Dearest, E ☑ **KU-519-245**

I hope you love this
book as Much as I
love you.

(Which is pretty Much
 near impossible becau-
 se I love you so Much)

With love
from Katy

♡ Happy ♡
 Birthday
     18.2.23

the
crystal
healer

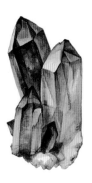

An Hachette UK Company
www.hachette.co.uk
First published in 2021 by Pyramid,
an imprint of Octopus Publishing Group Ltd
Carmelite House
50 Victoria Embankment
London, EC4Y 0DZ
www.octopusbooks.co.uk

ISBN: 978-0-7537-3462-9

A CIP catalogue record for this book is available from the British
Library

Printed and bound in China

10 9 8 7 6 5 4 3 2

Publisher: Lucy Pessell
Designer: Hannah Coughlin
Editor: Sarah Kennedy
Editorial Assistant: Emily Martin
Production Controller: Lisa Pinnell
Illustrations: Inna Sinano/Dreamstime.com; Natali Myasnikova/
Dreamstime.com

the
crystal
healer

Brenda Rosen

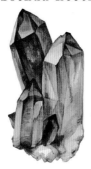

How to Use Crystals to
Heal Body and Mind

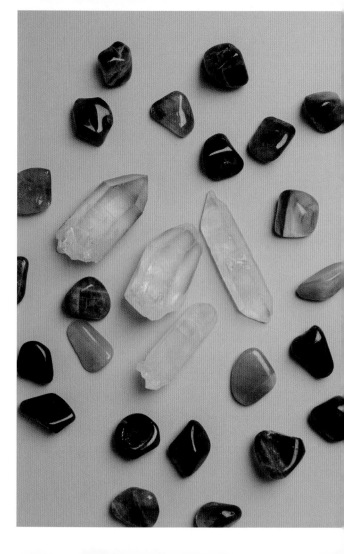

Contents

Introduction

Beautiful and mysterious, crystals have been used for thousands of years for decoration, adornment, protection and healing. Archaeologists have discovered beads, amulets, carvings and jewellery made of amber, jet, turquoise, lapis, garnet, carnelian, quartz and other crystals in excavations in every part of the world. Ancient people valued crystals for their magical and spiritual powers. Rulers wore rings and crowns set with precious gems. Shamans and healers used crystal amulets and gemstone remedies for healing and protection.

Crystals derive their power from the way they are created. The ancient belief that crystals are the bones of Mother Earth is not far from scientific truth. Millions of years ago, superheated gases and mineral solutions were forced upwards from the Earth's core towards the surface. As the molten rock gradually cooled, the mineral molecules formed orderly patterns.

The appearance of a crystal is affected by its mineral content, the temperature and pressure at which it formed and its rate of cooling. Hard and transparent crystals like diamonds were formed under tremendous heat and pressure. Softer stones such as calcite were created at lower temperatures.

Today we understand that the helpful properties of crystals arise from their structure. A crystal's molecules and atoms are arranged in a regular pattern that is repeated in exactly the same arrangement over and over in all directions. This orderly lattice-like structure gives crystals their unique ability to absorb, store, generate and transmit energy.

As you'll discover in this book, this ability allows crystals to be used to amplify, direct and balance the flow of life-force in your body and surroundings. You'll find that working with crystals is a gentle and natural way to improve your physical, emotional and spiritual wellbeing. This book is designed to offer you a wide variety of practical ways to use crystals to improve your health, balance your emotions and access spiritual peace and harmony.

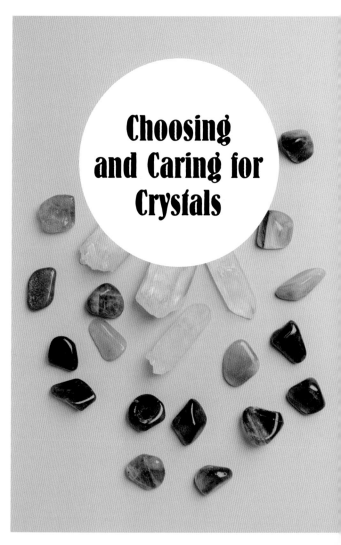

Choosing
and Caring for
Crystals

Crystal Qualities

Crystals can be classified in a number of ways, but the most useful qualities for practical purposes are a crystal's hardness, shape and colour.

Hardness

In 1812, German mineralogist Friedrich Mohs (1773–1839) ranked ten commonly available minerals in terms of how easily they could be scratched. The Mohs scale is still the accepted standard of crystal hardness. As you might expect, the diamond scores a 10 on the Mohs scale, while talc, which easily breaks up into common talcum powder, scores a 1. Other crystals fall somewhere in between.

Organic gemstones such as amber, coral and jet score 2.5–4. Lapis, opal and moonstone score between 5.5–6.5. Quartz, amethyst and gemstones such as emerald, sapphire and ruby score a 7 or above. Hardness is important when choosing crystals for healing and other practical purposes. Softer crystals can be used to absorb negative physical and emotional energy. It is the harder crystals that make the best choices for jewellery.

Shape

In their natural form, many crystals are rough, sharp or jagged – more like stones than translucent gems. Many of the small stones in crystal shops have been tumbled, a process that polishes a stone to enhance its colour and beauty. Polishing alters a crystal's appearance but does not affect its properties. A crystal's shape influences how it transmits energy.

Single-point crystals

These focus energy in a straight line. In general, pointed crystals are used to transmit energy or draw it off, depending on which way the point is facing. A symmetrical crystal wand is likely to have been artificially shaped.

Double-terminated crystals

These have a point on each end. Because they send and receive energy simultaneously, they are useful for balancing and integrating opposing forces, such as breaking up old patterns and overcoming addictions.

Crystal clusters

These radiate the energy of the crystal to the surrounding environment. They are useful for cleansing the energy in a room.

Geodes

These have a cave-like interior that holds and amplifies energy, releasing it slowly to their surroundings. They are a good choice for bedrooms, where a soothing flow of soft energy is beneficial.

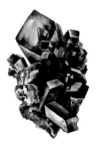

Colour

Perhaps the most important quality for crystal healing is colour. You have probably already experienced how colours affect your emotions – wearing a bright red sweater can make you feel sexy, while sitting in a room with cool blue walls is soothing and relaxing. In colour therapy, a form of complementary healing, the body is bathed in coloured light, or coloured crystals are placed directly on the body. Because of the links between the seven colours of the spectrum and your body's life-force, a crystal's colour energy can be assimilated into your body's energy field through your optic nerve or, as some believe, directly through your skin, transmitting or absorbing energy as needed for a healthy balance.

red crystals
such as bloodstone, red jasper, and carnelian increase your power, passion, courage and physical energy.

pink crystals
such as rose quartz, danburite and pink tourmaline foster kindness, love and compassion for yourself and others.

orange crystals
such as carnelian, fire opal and orange calcite enhance self-esteem, confidence and creativity.

yellow crystals
such as citrine, amber and sunstone aid self-expression and encourage optimism and positive attitudes.

green crystals
such as green fluorite and green aventurine soothe the emotions and promote harmony and balance.

blue crystals

such as blue lace agate, lapis and turquoise calm the mind, and cool and soothe the physical body.

purple crystals

such as amethyst, lepidolite and angelite help develop intuition and spiritual knowledge.

black crystals

such as smoky quartz, obsidian and labradorite are powerful protectors and help disperse negative energy and stress.

white or clear crystals

such as clear quartz, apophyllite and moonstone promote new beginnings, peace and tranquillity.

Choosing Crystals

Though the exercises in this book suggest particular crystals, choosing crystals should be personal and intuitive. You will find crystals have different voices and different personalities. The right crystals for you will draw your attention or your eye and ask to become part of your life.

Pick up a crystal that attracts you and hold it in your hands. Look at it from all angles and feel its weight, texture and shape. Tune in to the way the crystal feels in your hand. Close your eyes for a moment and see what you experience. You may feel a tingling on your skin or a sensation of warmth or coolness. You may also feel an energetic charge in some part of your body, such as the top of your head or the middle of your chest. If these sensations are pleasurable, the crystal you are holding is resonating with some aspect of your body-mind and is likely to be a good one for you to work with.

Looking after your crystals

Once you have chosen your crystals, look after them carefully. Crystals, especially those with unusual shapes such as points and clusters, can be fragile. To keep them safe, wrap each one separately in a silk scarf. Alternatively, find the right place in your home or office for each crystal, such as on your desk, on your bedside table or as part of an arrangement of houseplants near your favourite chair.

Though harder natural stones can scratch softer ones when they are stored together in a pouch, tumbled stones are, in general, more resistant to damage. It's perfectly fine to keep a collection of small tumbled stones in a silk bag or pouch.

Cleansing your crystals

Crystals that are used for healing or to balance the energy in your surroundings should be cleansed regularly. Cleansing your crystals when you first bring them home makes them uniquely yours. Cleansing them after each use rids them of negative energy and makes them ready to use again.

Some delicate crystals such as celestite or selenite can separate in water. Salt can damage other crystals, such as opals, changing their colour or making them appear dull or cloudy. If you are unsure about which cleansing method is best to use for a particular crystal, ask a knowledgeable dealer or choose one of these all-purpose methods.

Water and salt water

Hold a crystal that can be cleansed with water under a running tap, bathe it in water mixed with salt or immerse it in a natural water source such as a stream, waterfall or the sea. As the water flows over your crystal, hold the intention that all negative energy is being washed away and the crystal is being re-energized.

Smudging

All crystals can be cleansed by being surrounded by the smoke from a sage smudge stick. This method is especially useful for large crystals or for cleansing several crystals at once.

Moonlight

All crystals can also be cleansed by bathing them in the light of the moon for a few hours. Place a crystal on your windowsill or in your garden and allow the moonlight to draw off any impurities in order to recharge the crystal's energy.

General Guidelines

These guidelines about placing, wearing and carrying crystals and using gem essences will help you to get the most benefit from the crystal exercises in this book.

Placement on your body

Some of the crystal exercises in this book involve placing crystals on your chakra points or around your body. You'll find these most helpful when you are relaxed and uninterrupted, so close the door to your room, turn off your phone and give yourself permission to focus solely on yourself. Prepare a place where you will be comfortable lying on the floor, on a yoga mat or a folded blanket.

Wearing and carrying crystals

Crystal jewellery, such as pendants, rings or earrings, infuses you with continuous energy throughout your day. Also try carrying a crystal you are working with in a small silk pouch in your pocket or bag.

Gem essences

Gem essences have a subtle and gentle healing effect. They can be rubbed on an affected part of your body or poured into your bathwater.

How to prepare a simple gem essence

1. Place a cleansed crystal that can be immersed in water in a clean glass bowl filled with spring water. (If the crystal should not be immersed in water, place it in a small glass bowl and place the small bowl in a larger water-filled bowl.)

2. Place the bowl where it can stand in the sunlight for several hours.

3. Remove the crystal and pour the essence into a glass bottle with an airtight stopper. To keep an essence for more than a week, double the volume of the liquid in the bottle by adding clear alcohol or vodka as a preservative.

4. Label your essences with the crystal's name and the date of preparation. Store them in a cool, dark place.

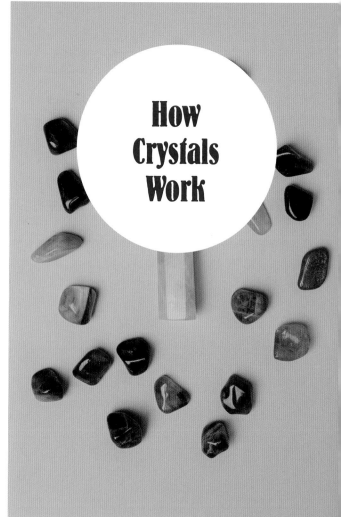

How Crystals Work

Crystals have a subtle but measurable 'vibration' or electromagnetic field, as does every object, including your body. The regularity of a crystal's structure makes this vibration especially coherent and helps crystals to transmit beneficial energy and absorb negative energy as needed to preserve a healthy balance.

Additionally, crystals may be so effective and popular because everyone responds emotionally to colours and to beautiful natural objects. Perhaps the good vibes you get from placing a stunning geode or crystal cluster on your desk are due both to the crystal's energy field and to your own positive emotional response to its radiant colour, striking shape and natural beauty.

Crystal healing may work in a similar way. Many of the healing exercises you'll find in this book ask you to pay attention to how you are feeling and then to take some action to relieve any problems, such as placing crystals in particular positions on your body or bathing in a gem essence. Paying attention to your body and emotions is always the first step to healing. In some cases, a crystal's vibration may simply help you to focus on your own potent healing.

Crystals and the Chakras

A type of healing called energy healing, which includes crystal therapy, is based on the idea that you can regulate your life energy by bringing attention to the body's seven energy centres, called the chakras. The chakras are swirling wheels of life energy aligned along the body's main energy channel, running parallel to the spine. Each chakra vibrates at a particular colour frequency and influences a particular set of physical, emotional and spiritual concerns.

Some of the techniques in this book are based on pairing crystals with the chakras. This handy chart will help you discover the body parts influenced by each chakra.

Crown Chakra

 Third Eye Chakra

 Throat Chakra

 Heart Chakra

 Solar Plexus Chakra

 Sacral Chakra

 Root Chakra

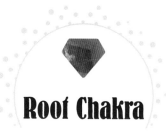

Root Chakra

related body parts	pelvis, bones, legs, ankles and feet, hips and rectum, immune system
potential health problems	sciatica, varicose veins, pelvic pain, rectal tumours, haemorrhoids, problems with hips, knees, ankles and feet
crystal colours	red, dark red, greenish-red, brownish-red, red-black
helpful crystals	smoky quartz, garnet, bloodstone, ruby, red jasper, red beryl, red calcite, red agate

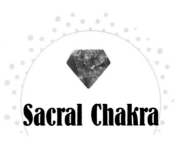

Sacral Chakra

related body parts	sexual organs, large intestine, kidney, bladder, appendix, lower spine
potential health problems	lower back pain, premenstrual tension, infertility, impotence, bladder infections, appendicitis, kidney stones
crystal colours	orange, reddish-orange, yellow-orange, orangey-brown, peach
helpful crystals	carnelian, orange calcite, citrine, tangerine quartz, fire opal, orange aragonite, moonstone

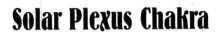

Solar Plexus Chakra

related body parts	stomach, liver, spleen, gallbladder, pancreas, small intestine, middle spine
potential health problems	ulcers, colon cancer, diabetes, indigestion, eating disorders, hepatitis, gallstones, constipation, diarrhoea
crystal colours	golden yellow, lemon yellow, honey-coloured, gold
helpful crystals	amber, yellow jasper, yellow tourmaline, golden topaz, tiger's eye, citrine, rutilated quartz, yellow calcite, sunstone

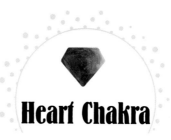

Heart Chakra

related body parts	heart and circulatory system, ribs, chest, lungs, shoulders and arms, breasts, upper spine
potential health problems	high blood pressure, heart disease, bronchitis, asthma, pneumonia, shoulder problems, breast cancer
crystal colours	pale pink, bright pink, rose pink, pale green, emerald green, bright green, olive green
helpful crystals	rose quartz, pink tourmaline, chrysophase, pink danburite, peridot, green fluorite, green aventurine, green citrine, jade

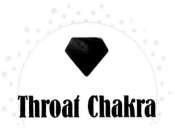

Throat Chakra

related body parts	throat, neck, mouth, teeth, gums, jaw, thyroid, neck vertebrae, oesophagus
potential health problems	sore throat, laryngitis, frequent colds, gum disease, dental problems, thyroid problems, swollen glands, stiff neck
crystal colours	turquoise blue, light blue, blue-green, bright blue, powder blue, royal blue
helpful crystals	turquoise, lapis lazuli, aquamarine, blue lace agate, celestite, blue sapphire, sodalite, aqua aura

Third Eye Chakra

related body parts	brain, central nervous system, eyes, ears, nose, sinuses, pituitary gland, pineal gland
potential health problems	epilepsy, eye problems, sinus infections, headaches, migraine, stroke, deafness, insomnia, nightmares
crystal colours	deep purple, purple-blue, dark lavender
helpful crystals	amethyst, iolite, azurite, purple fluorite lilac kunzite, electric blue obsidian, sugilite, blue chalcedony

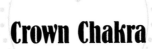

Crown Chakra

related body parts	whole body systems: skeletal system, muscular system, skin, neurological system
potential health problems	chronic exhaustion without physical cause, skin diseases, environmental illness, neurosis, mental illness
crystal colours	pale lilac, lavender, violet, clear, snow white, translucent
helpful crystals	purple jasper, purple sapphire, lilac danburite, labradorite (spectorolite), clear quartz, apophyllite, diamond

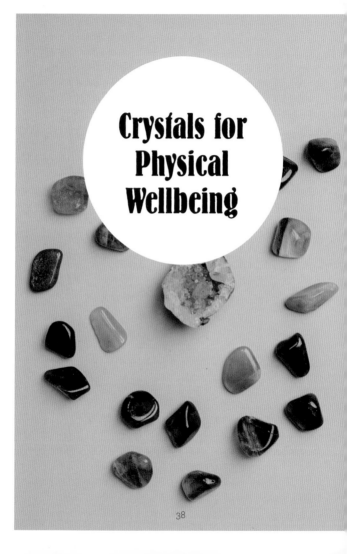

Crystals for Physical Wellbeing

The theory behind crystal healing is simple. Crystals are superb energy transmitters. Their crystalline structure amplifies your healing intentions and restores and rebalances your body's energy by removing blockages, drawing off excess energy and shoring up weaknesses. Crystal healing is not a substitute for traditional medical care, but it can help in many practical ways. Healing with crystals also empowers you to take personal responsibility for your health, using simple, natural methods. The crystal exercises in this section will teach you how to treat common physical ailments.

Pain Relief

Pain anywhere in your body is a message that something is wrong. The discomfort may be due to a physical illness or it may reflect emotional or spiritual distress. Crystal healing is most effective when you take the time to investigate all possible reasons for your discomfort, keeping in mind that the cause may be a combination of factors.

Exercise: quartz pain relief

For this exercise you will need one smoky quartz crystal with a single termination point and one clear quartz crystal with a single termination point. Single-point crystals focus energy or draw it off, depending on which way the point is facing.

1. Lie down on a yoga mat or folded blanket or sit comfortably on the floor.

2. Hold the smoky quartz crystal in your left hand with the termination pointing away from the painful area. Move the crystal in a small circle just above the painful area in an anticlockwise motion. As you circle the crystal, breathe into the painful area, carrying with your breath the intention to release the pain. In your mind's eye, imagine the crystal is a sponge drawing off and absorbing any painful or blocked energy.

3. When the pain has decreased, switch hands and crystals. Hold the clear quartz crystal in your right hand with the termination pointing towards the area being healed. Move the crystal in a small circle just above the area in a clockwise motion. As you circle the crystal, imagine that the crystal is releasing natural life-force energy to revitalize and restore your body's optimum energy balance.

Nasal Congestion

The nasal congestion you get with a common cold is generally caused by a respiratory virus. Though crystal therapy cannot prevent you from catching a cold, it can help to alleviate your symptoms and make you more comfortable. Of course, you should also follow medical advice, including getting plenty of rest and drinking hot tea and other liquids to keep your body hydrated while it heals.

Exercise: crystal steam inhalation

Inhaling steam fused with a gem essence can relieve the stuffy nose and sinus congestion of a cold or flu. For this technique you will need a small piece of sodalite or blue lace agate.

1. Make a gem essence with a sodalite or blue lace agate crystal (see page 25 for instructions).

2. Half-fill a bowl with boiling water. Pour the gem essence into the bowl. Bend over the bowl and cover your head with a towel.

3. Breathe in the gem essence-infused steam deeply through your nose for several minutes. If you are nursing a cold or flu at home, it's fine to repeat this technique up to five times a day.

4. In the evening, pour more of the gem essence into your bathwater and relax as you inhale the healing steam.

Sore Throat

The throat chakra, which influences the throat, neck and mouth, vibrates at the frequency of blue light. So the best crystal for ills affecting your throat, such as a sore throat, laryngitis, swollen glands or hoarseness due to a cold or flu, is blue lace agate. This lovely powdery or periwinkle blue stone, often banded with white lacy threads, harmonizes perfectly with the energy of the throat chakra, activating it to help soothe and calm a painful throat.

Exercise: crystal gargle

For this technique you will need one tumbled blue lace agate crystal.

1. Half-fill a bowl with spring water.

2. Immerse a cleansed blue lace agate crystal in the water. Place the bowl on the windowsill, preferably overnight, when the crystal can absorb energy from the light of the moon. If that timing is not convenient, set the bowl aside for at least eight hours.

3. Remove the crystal and gargle with the gem essence-infused water. If you are nursing a

sore throat at home, gargle with this gem essence every two hours as needed.

Digestion

Your digestive system includes the oesophagus, stomach and intestines, as well as the organs that produce substances that help break down the food you eat, such as the liver, pancreas and gallbladder.

Digestion is under the influence of the solar plexus chakra, located at the abdomen above the navel. Radiating golden-yellow fire energy, this is like an inner sun, fuelling not only digestion but also your vitality, drive and passion. When it is functioning well, life energy shines outwards from your body's core, helping you get nourishment from both food and life experiences. When it is out of balance, you may feel irritable, angry or resentful and have a tendency to blame others when things go wrong. Not surprisingly, you may also experience stomach aches and other digestive upsets.

Exercise: citrine inner sun meditation

For this meditation you will need one piece of citrine. A small polished stone, a point or a geode work equally well.

1. Sit comfortably cross-legged on the floor or on a chair with your feet flat on the ground. Be sure that your back is straight. Close your eyes.

2. Hold the piece of citrine with your hands resting comfortably against your abdomen.

3. Breathe slowly and deeply, taking air all the way down to your belly. As you breathe

in, imagine that the citrine crystal in your hands is shining like the sun, energizing with its golden light the inner sun of your solar plexus chakra.

4. As you breathe out, imagine that the warming and invigorating energy of your inner sun is spreading throughout your body, strengthening your digestive system, healing its ills and filling you with vitality, warmth and passion.

Hormonal Imbalance

Many women experience their menstrual cycles as natural and easy. Others have problems with infertility, painful or irregular menstruation, and hot flushes and other uncomfortable symptoms after menopause. Lifestyle choices, including a nurturing diet, regular exercise, maintaining an appropriate weight, avoiding addictions such as smoking and alcohol and reducing stress can help regulate hormones. When problems do occur, crystal therapy is one of the ways a woman can focus self-healing attention on her natural cycles and rebalance the flow of energy through her reproductive organs.

Exercise: moonstone rebalance

For this exercise you will need one tumbled moonstone crystal. Because the monthly phases of the moon mirror a woman's natural cycles, moonstone is nurturing to the female reproductive system.

1. Sit comfortably cross-legged on the floor or on a chair with your feet flat on the floor. Make sure that you keep your back straight.

2. Breathe gently and smoothly in a regular rhythm.

3. Hold the moonstone crystal gently in your hands in front of you.

4. Allow your soft gaze to caress its translucent white or creamy iridescent shimmering curves.

5. Remind yourself that, just like the moon, your reproductive system waxes and wanes in naturally recurring cycles.

6. As the gentle feminine energy of the moonstone rebalances and strengthens your reproductive processes, allow your heart to open in appreciation of the beauty of your own moon-like rhythms.

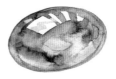

Immune System

Your immune system helps your body stay healthy. Its interconnected network of glands and organs stimulates the production of lymphocytes, a type of white blood cell that seeks out and destroys disease-causing viruses and bacteria. It also eliminates waste from the food you eat and the air you breathe. Two important parts of your immune system are the thymus, a butterfly-shaped gland in the centre of your chest, and the spleen, a purplish-red organ on the upper left side of your abdomen.

Exercise: immune system stimulator

For this exercise you will need one aqua aura quartz point and one clear quartz tumbled crystal.

1. Lie down on a yoga mat or folded blanket. Place a flat pillow under your head to ease any tension in your neck.

2. Place the aqua aura point on your thymus and the tumbled clear quartz crystal in the centre of your forehead.

3. Leave the aqua aura and quartz crystals in place and remain still for 10–20 minutes.

Detox

Detoxification means helping your body cleanse itself of the residues of living in the modern world, including toxins from air and water pollution, food additives, cigarette smoke and other environmental hazards.

Crystal therapy can help to support natural detoxification, strengthening your immune system. In the technique described overleaf, you use a crystal to apply gentle pressure to the palms of your hands. In reflexology, the palms of the hands and soles of the feet are regarded as mirroring the whole body. Stimulating your palms sends energy through the pathways of your body, clearing blockages and encouraging your body to release toxins.

Exercise: danburite detox

For this exercise you will need one natural danburite crystal with a single termination. A powerful healing stone, danburite strengthens the liver and gallbladder, supporting detoxification.

1. Sit comfortably. Hold the danburite crystal in your right hand.
2. Gently circle the crystal into the palm of your left hand, running the termination point of the crystal over the whole palm from the tips

of each finger to the wrist. Don't push hard or dig the crystal into your hand. Simply move the danburite over your skin in a rhythmic motion.

3. Switch the crystal into your left hand and repeat the process, running the crystal over the whole of your right palm.

4. When you have finished, wash your hands and drink at least 250 ml (8 fl oz) of spring water Also, be sure to cleanse the crystal.

Improving Sleep

Many people have difficulties falling asleep or staying asleep. Sometimes the problem is caused by stress or by drinking excessive amounts of coffee or alcohol. Keeping a sleep diary can help you become aware of behaviour patterns that may be disturbing your sleep. You can also use a journal to keep track of how well the crystal therapy technique described below works for you. Review your entries regularly and make changes in your routine to see whether they improve your sleep.

Exercise: crystal therapy for insomnia

For this technique you will need one tumbled amethyst or one tumbled sodalite crystal. Amethyst is a natural tranquillizer that helps to calm and soothe the mind.

1. Lie comfortably on your back in bed. Place the amethyst or sodalite crystal on your brow chakra. Leave the crystal in place as you practise one of the following relaxation techniques. It's fine to leave the crystal in place as you fall asleep. Or, if you prefer, remove it after 15 minutes and put it under your pillow.

2. Put a hand on your stomach and take long, slow breaths, allowing your belly to expand as you inhale. As you exhale, relax your chest and shoulders. Focus your attention on the rise and fall of your abdomen until you feel that you are completely relaxed.

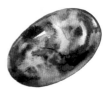

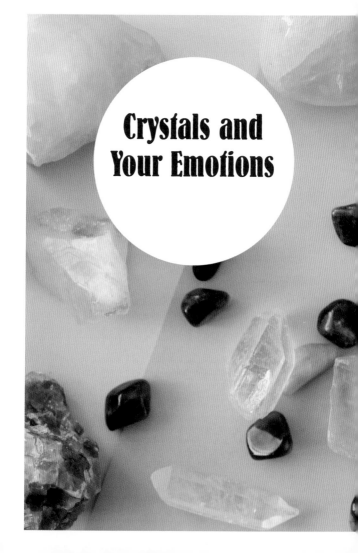

Crystals and
Your Emotions

You've no doubt had days when everything seems to go wrong and your emotional reactions are way over the top. You may be so upset that you can't stop crying, or you may find yourself snapping at your kids or colleagues, or you may feel so worked up that you can barely think straight.

Because they work on the mind and body energetically, crystals are especially helpful in overcoming mental and emotional problems. From time to time the flow of life-force through the chakras can become unbalanced and emotional problems may indicate that either too much or too little energy is travelling through a chakra. Your own experience is likely to confirm this idea. Think of how constricted your heart feels when you are lonely or how much fiery energy you feel in your solar plexus when you are angry. Crystals help you to balance the flow of your energy and improve your mental and emotional health. Because of their soothing and balancing effect on all levels of your being, they can help your body slow the release of stress hormones, increase your awareness of negative thought patterns and mental attitudes and quieten your emotional responses. In this section, you will find exercises to help you take care of your emotions.

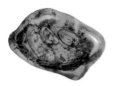

Stress

When you are stressed your adrenal glands are secreting a hormone that is spreading throughout your body, raising your blood pressure, speeding up your heart and causing the 'on alert' feeling that is often called the 'fight or flight' response. This natural reaction is your body's way of providing the extra energy that you need to protect yourself from danger. However, when being on alert turns into a regular habit, your body's energy reserves become depleted.

Exercise: crystal pairs

For this exercise you will need a pair of crystals, depending on your situation and needs. The first crystal mentioned in each pair overleaf is the more active and energetic stone. Its job is to relieve stress. The second crystal calms and soothes. Palm stones – round, flat stones that sit comfortably in your hand – are especially good for this exercise, but you can also use small tumbled stones.

Crystal Pairings:

Amber and blue chalcedony
Amber absorbs negative energy, while blue chalcedony promotes acceptance and optimism.

Clear quartz and amethyst
Clear quartz relieves pain and tension, while amethyst brings calmness and mental clarity.

Tiger's eye and aragonite
Tiger's eye slows the release of stress hormones, while aragonite encourages insight into the causes of your distress.

1. Choose one of the crystal pairs opposite. Sit comfortably or lie on your back on a yoga mat or folded blanket.

2. Hold the more active crystal (the first crystal in each pair) in your dominant hand (the hand you write with) and hold the calming crystal in your receptive hand.

3. Close your eyes. Consciously relax your muscles, starting with your feet and working your way up your body. Allow about 20 minutes for the crystals to do their work.

Anxiety and Depression

When you are anxious about something, you may feel as if your thoughts are no longer under your control. Your mind circles round and round the same track, repeating a pattern of uneasy thoughts and mental pictures. Persistent worry can negatively impact on your physical health as well as your emotional wellbeing. You may develop headaches and muscle pain, or you may have trouble sleeping. Without relief, you may eventually become depressed. Cultures around the world have used crystals to release the nervous tension that accompanies worry.

Exercise: worry relief web

For this exercise you will need two natural kunzite crystals and five tumbled lepidolite crystals.

1. Lie down on a yoga mat or folded blanket. Place a flat pillow under your head to ease any tension in your neck.
2. Place one kunzite above your head and one kunzite between your feet.
3. Place the lepidolite crystals on your brow, throat, heart, solar plexus and sacral chakras.

4.   Follow your breathing all the way in and all the way out for 20 minutes while the crystals help to discharge the stuck emotional energy of obsessive worry.

Fears and Phobias

Feeling fearful when you are in actual danger is part of your body's natural self-protection mechanism. Feeling apprehensive before you give a speech or visit the dentist is also natural, so long as you are able to control your fear and keep going. But when fear interferes with your ability to enjoy life fully, it may be a reason for concern.

An intense, irrational fear of a situation or object is called a phobia. Common phobias include fear of closed-in places, heights, tunnels, lifts, water, flying and spiders! Phobias get in the way of daily living by redirecting your life energy towards avoiding the thing you fear. They can also cause physical symptoms, such as stomach cramps or light-headedness.

Exercise: releasing fears and phobias

For this exercise you will need one aquamarine crystal with a single termination and/or one smoky quartz crystal with a single termination. Aquamarine (technique 1) brings courage and calms your mind. Smoky quartz (technique 2) helps keep your body grounded in fearful situations.

Technique 1

1. Sit comfortably cross-legged on the floor or on a chair with your feet flat on the floor. Place the crystals nearby. Close your eyes and follow your breathing all the way in and all the way out until you feel both centred and relaxed.

2. With the fingers of your right hand, tap your breastbone three times between your heart and your throat. This place is the witness point.

3. Hold the aquamarine to your witness point with the termination towards your head. Think about the fear or phobia you want to release. You may feel tingling or throbbing in your witness point as your mind becomes calm.

Technique 2

In Step 3, hold the smoky quartz to your witness point with the termination towards your lap (downwards). Think about the fear or phobia you want to release. You may feel tingling or throbbing in your witness point as your fear is released and body becomes more grounded and centred.

Anger

Anger feels awful. Your face turns red, your heart races and it hurts to breathe. Anger is often hot and raging. It can make you yell or throw things or pound your fist on the table. It can also manifest as passive-aggressive behaviour and coldly calculated strategies to get back at someone who has hurt you.

Ironically, anger often hurts you as much as it hurts the person towards whom it is directed. The Buddha described anger as reaching your hand into the fire to pick up a hot coal to throw at someone else. Of course, your hand gets burned first! Crystals can help you to release your angry feelings before they cause you damage.

Exercise: release and forgiveness

For this exercise you will need one apophyllite, amethyst or lapis lazuli crystal. Try all three and see which works best for you.

1. Sit comfortably cross-legged on the floor and place the crystal you have selected nearby.

2. Bring to mind the image of the person or situation towards which your anger is directed. Say, either in your mind or out loud, why you feel resentment, hurt or anger.

3. Pick up the crystal and hold it in your hands. Say, either in your mind or out loud, that in the past you have felt anger towards this person or situation, but now you are going to do your best to release it.

4. Say words of release such as: 'I release my anger and forgive you.' As you do, imagine that the anger is draining away, leaving your mind and body at peace.

Brain Fog

Daily life provides many examples of the close connection between your emotions and your mental processes. On days when you are depressed or your self-confidence is low, your mind may feel sluggish or confused, or it may skip restlessly from one topic to another. It may be hard to focus and you may forget appointments or be unable to finish tasks and meet deadlines. Crystals can help to calm an overactive mind and clear confusion.

Exercise: mind support layout

For this exercise you will need one tumbled sodalite, one natural clear quartz, one polished labradorite, one tumbled amethyst and one tumbled or natural smoky quartz.

1. Lie down on a yoga mat or folded blanket. Place a flat pillow under your head to ease tension in your neck.

2. Place the amethyst crystal above the top of your head.

3. Place the sodalite crystal high on your forehead. Use a piece of tape to keep it in place, if necessary.

4. Place the quartz in between your eyebrows.

5. Place the labradorite to the right of your head.

6. Place the smoky quartz to the left of your head and spend 20 minutes lying quietly with the crystals in place, focusing on your breathing.

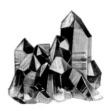

Sex and Relationships

The sacral chakra governs sexuality and blockages here can make it hard for you to feel desire. A well-functioning sacral chakra opens you to the joys of touching and being touched, of giving and receiving, of achieving sexual satisfaction and enjoying the sensation of giving satisfaction to others. Orange-coloured crystals, such as carnelian, orange calcite and citrine, vibrate with the energy of the sacral chakra, releasing blockages and encouraging the free flow of sexual energy.

Exercise: sacral pleasure breath

For this exercise you will need one or two pieces of orange carnelian, orange calcite or citrine.

1. Prepare a private place to work in that's warm enough for you to be comfortable without clothes. If you wish, use candles, flowers, soft music and pillows to make the space more intimate and relaxing.

2. Take off your clothes and lie down on a yoga mat or folded blanket. Place a flat pillow under your head to ease any tension in your neck.

3. Place the orange-coloured crystal on your sacral chakra, just below your navel.

4. As you breathe in, visualize the air coming in through your nose and travelling down your body, carrying warmth and energy to your lower abdomen. Visualize or feel a vibrant orange glow flowing from the crystal into your sacral chakra, awakening and healing your sexual centre. You should continue the visualization for 5–15 minutes.

Heartache

If you have been hurt in your relationships, you may have closed down the flow of energy through your heart chakra to protect yourself from being hurt again. Opening to unhappy memories is sometimes painful, but it is a necessary first step to getting your emotional energy moving again.

The crystal healing meditation opposite combines the energies of three crystals that gently release past hurts and heal and balance your emotions.

Exercise: heartache relief circle

For this exercise you will need six tumbled amethyst crystals, six blue lace agate crystals and one natural kunzite crystal. Sit comfortably on the floor, using a pillow for support if you wish.

1. Alternate the blue lace agate and amethyst in a circle around you.

2. Hold the kunzite against your heart chakra, using both hands. Bring to mind the past hurt you wish to heal. Imagine or feel that the kunzite is gently drawing out the painful emotional energy of this experience and replacing it with tenderness and compassion for your past suffering.

3. When you feel ready, hold the kunzite away from your body, pointing it outwards beyond the crystal circle. In your mind, or out loud, speak words of release, such as 'I release myself from dwelling on the past.' Imagine or feel that your anger and sadness are leaving you and travelling far away.

4. When you feel that this part of the process is complete, place the kunzite on the floor outside the crystal circle. Now imagine that your mind and body are bathed in the healing vibrations of the crystals surrounding you. Try

to absorb this healing energy. In your mind or out loud, say words of comfort and hope, such as 'I open my heart to new possibilities.' As you do, feel that your emotions are calm and balanced and that your mind is at peace.

Opening the Heart

Rose quartz has a strong energetic connection to the heart chakra. Often called the stone of unconditional love, it encourages healthy self-love, forgiveness and reconciliation and opens the heart to romantic love. Rose quartz is also a comforting stone when you have suffered heartbreak or loss.

Exercise: heart rose meditation

This meditation will allow love to flow into your being and open you to all the possibilities of romance. You will need one polished rose quartz crystal.

1. Lie on your back on a yoga mat or blanket. Place a flat pillow under your head to ease any tension in your neck.

2. Place the rose quartz heart on your heart chakra, in the centre of your chest.

3. Spend a few minutes watching your breath, paying attention to the expansion and contraction of your chest. Listen to your heartbeat.

4. Bring to mind the image of someone you love or have loved strongly in your life. Appreciate as fully as you can everything that was or is wonderful about this relationship.

5. Now turn your attention to your heart chakra. Visualize it as a beautiful budding rose being warmed by the gentle vibrations of the rose quartz heart. Allow the tender feelings you have for the loved person you are recalling to slowly open the petals of the rosebud until your heart rose is in full and glorious bloom.

Protection on the Go

Healthy emotional balance also depends on living in a safe and protected environment. Emotionally sensitive people are often prone to 'picking up' stress, anger and other negative emotions from the people around them. If you commute on public transport, for instance, you may absorb negative emotional energy from literally hundreds of strangers before you even get to work. Many people are also sensitive to the electromagnetic pollution generated by computers, mobile phones and other appliances. Crystals can help you surround yourself with a bubble of safety and protection at home, at work and when you're on the go.

Exercise: on the go pouch

Create a crystal protection pouch to keep you safe wherever you go.

Choose one or more small tumbled stones from each of the following groups of crystals:

- To cleanse and transform negative energy: amber, bloodstone or smoky quartz
- To attract calm and peaceful energy: amethyst, kunzite or rose quartz
- To protect against electromagnetic pollution: clear quartz, fluorite or sodalite
- For personal protection: aqua aura, carnelian or labradorite

Place the crystals in a small silk pouch and carry it in your pocket or bag. You can also place it on your bedside table or under your pillow while you sleep.

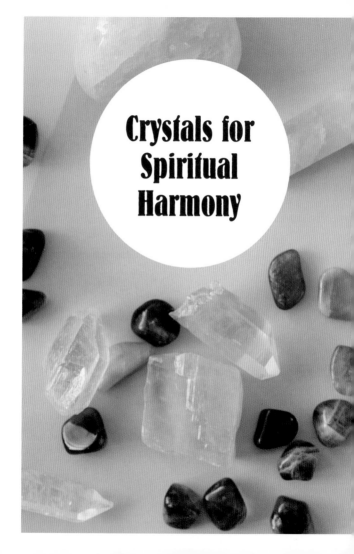

Crystals for Spiritual Harmony

Crystals have been valued since ancient times as aids to vision, intuition, wisdom and other psychic and spiritual gifts. As you will discover in this chapter, working with crystals can help you develop these qualities in yourself.

Because of their unique ability to focus and transmit psychic energy, crystals can strengthen your natural spiritual abilities. A crystal's spiritual power is enhanced by your motivation and intention. If you seek inner balance, crystals can help you align your body's energies. If you wish to create harmony in your environment, crystals can make your home a peaceful sanctuary. Holding a crystal during meditation helps you sharpen your intuition, enlarge your creative vision and deepen your ability to concentrate. Placed under your pillow with intention, crystals can open you to dreams that provide spiritual guidance and personal insight. This section is filled with exercises to help you fully engage with the spiritual elements of your mind and body.

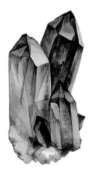

Balance Your Chakras

Though you may not be able to see your chakras with your physical eyes, you can use your intuition to sense them. When you feel unwell or your emotions are out of control, turn your attention within and see what you can sense about your chakras. Focus your inner sight on each chakra in turn, starting with the root chakra. If you sense a variation in the size, spin or colour of one of your chakras – for instance, a throat chakra that is pale rather than vivid blue, or a solar plexus chakra that has too little energy or seems to be spinning too slowly – use this colour balancing technique to strengthen the chakra's energy.

Exercise: chakra colour balance

As you will have read earlier on in this book, each chakra corresponds to one of the colours in the light spectrum. Crystals that vibrate at a similar colour frequency can help to regularize the chakra's spin and bring it back into alignment.

1. Consult the chakra chart on pages 30-37 and choose a crystal that corresponds in colour to the chakra that you wish to strengthen.
2. Sit comfortably cross-legged on the floor or on a chair with your feet flat on the floor. Be sure that your back is straight. Breathe gently and smoothly in a regular rhythm.
3. Hold the crystal you have chosen in your hands. Visualize the coloured light and energy of the crystal radiating out and flowing into your chakra, balancing and strengthening its energy. Maintain a state of relaxed awareness for 5–10 minutes.

Enhance Intuition

The 'voices' that you hear and the 'visions' that you see when you go inside to access your intuition are, in fact, part of you. They reflect the understanding you have gained from everything that you have experienced in your life – even things you have forgotten or never consciously knew.

Quietening your everyday mind creates the space for the deep wisdom of your mind to provide inspiration and guidance. Using a crystal sphere as a focus point is a time-honoured method of accessing this wisdom.

Exercise: crystal gazing

For this exercise you will need a sphere of clear quartz, obsidian or smoky quartz and a small white candle.

1. Light the candle and dim the lights in the room. Hold the crystal sphere in your cupped hands for several moments and focus on your breathing, continuing until you feel relaxed and centred.

2. As you hold the sphere, clarify your intention. If you are seeking the answer to a question, state it in words. If you are seeking guidance about a situation, phrase what you wish to know in a clear, positive, open-ended way. For instance, 'I wish to understand Jack better to improve our relationship' or 'I need guidance about setting appropriate boundaries for my daughter.'

3. Place the sphere in front of you with the burning candle behind it.

4. Gaze at the crystal with half-closed eyes and allow images to form in your mind and on the sphere. Follow any images that appear until you have learned everything that you can.

5. When you feel that the process is complete, acknowledge what you have discovered as the deep wisdom of your own intuition. Wrap the crystal sphere in a cloth and blow out the candle.

Psychic Gifts

With practice and good intentions, anyone can develop psychic gifts such as clairvoyance and telepathy to some degree. Used with integrity and the proper motivation, these gifts can help you extend your mind and senses beyond the horizons of time and space and discover information that is helpful for you and others.

One of the most powerful crystals for developing your psychic gifts is moldavite. This strange crystal is said to be of extra-terrestrial origin. It was formed about 15 million years ago when a meteor collided with Earth in the Moldau river valley in the Czech Republic. Combining the energies of Earth and the heavens, moldavite encourages psychic and spiritual growth.

Exercise: moldavite journey

For this exercise you will need one piece of moldavite.

1. Lie down on a yoga mat or folded blanket. Place a flat pillow under your head to ease tension in your neck.

2. Place the moldavite crystal on your brow chakra.

3. Close your eyes and focus on your breathing for a few moments until you feel relaxed and centred. Clarify your intention. Decide where you would like to journey to and what you wish to discover, and consider how this information might be of help to you and others.

4. Allow an image to form in your mind's eye of the place to which you wish to journey to. Allow yourself to enter the story, like stepping across the frame into a picture, knowing that you can return instantly any time you wish.

5. Allow the story to unfold as long as feels right. With gratitude for what you have discovered, end by taking a deep breath. Open your eyes and stretch your arms and legs. Roll gently to one side and sit up.

Meditation

Many people misunderstand the goal of meditation. Meditation is not a passive activity, and although relaxing your body and calming your mind are among its benefits, they are not its central purpose. The aim of meditation is focused awareness – a state of being more present to yourself.

One useful way to think about meditation is as a form of clear internal communication. As you quieten your body and mind and look inside yourself, you become aware that your perceptions, emotions, thoughts and beliefs, including beliefs about yourself such as 'I have a bad temper' or 'I can't manage money', are not permanent and unchanging. Instead, they come and go, like clouds passing across the sky.

Exercise: blue sky meditation

For this exercise you will need one blue-coloured crystal, such as a piece of polished turquoise or lapis lazuli. As you will have read earlier on, blue crystals open the throat chakra, encouraging clarity and self-awareness.

1.   Sit comfortably on a cushion or a chair with your feet flat on the floor. Hold the turquoise or lapis lazuli crystal to your throat for a few moments. Imagine that you are inhaling the bright blue energy of the crystal, relaxing your throat and enhancing your ability to

communicate truthfully with yourself. Then relax and hold the crystal gently in your lap.

2. Bring to awareness whatever thoughts or emotions are passing through your mind at this moment. Do not follow these thoughts or feelings. Simply observe them. Accept whatever arises in your mind.

3. Allow the thought to arise that your mind is like a crystalline blue sky – perhaps the colour of the crystal you are holding. All the thoughts and feelings that pass through your mind are like clouds that move across the sky, coming into view and then passing away. Remind yourself that these passing clouds are not your mind. Your mind is like the sky – vast, clear, empty and filled with light.

4. Focus on the clear blue sky of mind beyond all thoughts and feelings for 10–20 minutes, or until you feel relaxed, aware and at peace.

Spiritual Connection

Crystals with a high vibration, such as selenite, angelite and celestite, stimulate the higher chakras, lifting you to an awareness of universal consciousness – the realm in which you are simultaneously uniquely yourself and yet one with everything that is. Connecting with this level of being regularly has the power to transform your life. You realize that you are much more than your physical body and your mind. Like a crystal, you are essentially light energy that has been slowed down or frozen into physical form. Meditation gives your inner light a chance to shine.

Exercise: inner light meditation

For this exercise you will need one piece of angelite, celestite or selenite.

1.   Sit comfortably cross-legged on the floor or on a chair with your feet flat on the floor. Allow your eyes to close and take a few conscious breaths, following your breathing all the way in and all the way out.

2.   Hold the crystal you have chosen above the top of your head for a few moments. Then relax and hold it gently in your lap.

3.   Visualize that the crystal you held above your head has left behind a sphere of pure transparent white light. Spend a few moments focusing on the presence of this light. Don't worry if the sphere does not appear clearly. It's fine just to have a sense that it is there.

4.   Imagine that this sphere of light represents every wonderful quality that you have ever wished for: compassion, generosity, patience, enthusiasm, wisdom – the complete fulfilment of your highest potential.

5.   Imagine now that the sphere of light decreases in size, shrinking until it becomes the size of

a bird's egg, about 2.5 cm (1 inch) in diameter. Imagine that this sphere enters your body through your crown chakra and descends to your heart chakra, bringing these qualities into your heart.

6. Imagine now the sphere of light expands once more, slowly filling your entire body. As it does, feel that your physical parts, your perceptions, emotions, thoughts and beliefs are dissolving into light, becoming what they are in essence – pure formless energy.

7. Remain in this serene and joyful state as long as you wish.

Dreams

Like meditation, dreams allow you to travel beneath the busy surface of consciousness to the depths where currents of insight and understanding flow. Grounding stones such as red jasper and bloodstone stimulate dreaming. Crystals with a higher vibration, such as amethyst, danburite and moonstone, can help you recall and decode dream messages.

Exercise: crystal dreaming

For this exercise you will need one piece of red jasper or bloodstone, and one piece of amethyst, celestite, danburite or moonstone.

1. Before you go to sleep, place the bloodstone or red jasper under your pillow. Place a notebook and pen near your bed. Allow your last thought before falling asleep to be your intention to dream vividly and to remember your dreams.

2. When you wake, lie still and bring your dreams to mind. Write notes about everything you remember.

3. Later, set aside some time to decode your dreams. Seat yourself comfortably. Place your notebook in your lap and hold the amethyst, celestite, danburite or moonstone crystal in your hands. Close your eyes and breathe in the energy of the crystal until you feel centred and relaxed.

4. Begin by making associations. Assume that every person, place, colour, sound, situation and event in your dream is trying to tell you something. Write down every association you can for each image. An association is any feeling, word, memory or idea that pops up in response to an image.

5. Next, make personal connections. Look over your list of associations and decide which associations 'click' – that is, which spontaneously bring up energy or strong feelings. For each, ask yourself: What part of me is that? What do I have in common with that? Where have I seen that in my life? Make notes about what you discover.

6. Finally, find the message. Use your intuition to draw the associations and connections together into a unified picture. Ask yourself: What message is this dream trying to communicate? What changes is it advising me to make? Don't expect the message to be clear immediately. You'll know you are on the right track when an interpretation gives you a surge of energy.

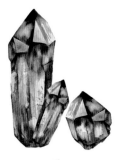